Narjes Karmous

Hysterosalpingography versus hysteroscopy for infertility

Narjes Karmous

Hysterosalpingography versus hysteroscopy for infertility

Performance in diagnosing intrauterine anomalies

ScienciaScripts

Imprint

Cover image: www.ingimage.com

This book is a translation from the original published under ISBN 978-620-6-73041-5.

Publisher:
Sciencia Scripts
is a trademark of
Dodo Books Indian Ocean Ltd. and OmniScriptum S.R.L publishing group

120 High Road, East Finchley, London, N2 9ED, United Kingdom
Str. Armeneasca 28/1, office 1, Chisinau MD-2012, Republic of Moldova, Europe
Managing Directors: Ieva Konstantinova, Victoria Ursu
info@omniscriptum.com

Printed at: see last page
ISBN: 978-620-8-63332-5

INTRODUCTION

According to the World Health Organisation (WHO), infertility is defined as the inability achieve pregnancy after twelve months or more regular unprotected sexual intercourse (1). According to recent WHO global statistics, the infertility rate has been estimated at 17.5% of the adult population (2).Uterine pathologies are responsible for 15% of female infertility (3). These anomalies include endometrial polyps, leiomyomas, intrauterine synechiae and congenital uterine malformations such as septate uterus (4).Pelvic ultrasound, hydro sonography, hysterosalpingography (HSG) and hysteroscopy (HSC) are the accepted procedures for exploring the uterine cavity in cases of infertility. At present, pelvic ultrasound and HSG are recommended as procedures, and hysteroscopy is recommended if an abnormality is found (5). HSG is a safe, simple and inexpensive procedure which enables the patency of the uterine cavity and fallopian tubes to be explored. However, this examination involves radiation and is not always accessible in Tunisia (6). HSC is considered the gold standard, as it provides a direct view of the uterine cavity. According to the International Society for Gynecologic Endoscopy and the literature, diagnostic hysteroscopy is the reference examination for diagnosing endometrial and intracavitary pathologies (7,8,9), and can therefore be used to diagnose discrete changes in the uterine cavity. It also has the advantage of enabling biopsies and therapeutic measures to be taken. On the other hand, it is a more invasive procedure (6). The data in the literature is controversial as to the superiority of one technique over the other as a first-line examination. In fact, some studies consider that these two techniques are mandatory in infertility work-up, others consider that in the case of a normal HSG, the indication for HSC is no longer there, while other studies recommend that HSG no longer has a place in the infertility (6). In Tunisia, there is a lack of data on this subject. The aim of our study was to compare HSG data with those from HSC in patients being investigated for infertility, in order compare the performance of the two techniques in exploring the uterine cavity.

METHODS

1. TYPE OF STUDY, LOCATION AND PERIOD

This was a retrospective, longitudinal, monocentric and comparative study carried out in department B of obstetrics and gynaecology at Charles Nicolle Hospital in Tunis, extending over 7 years and 10 months, from 1 January 2016 to 31 October 2024, and including patients being monitored for infertility who had undergone HSG and HSC.

2. POPULATION STUDIED

During the study period and while respecting anonymity, we compiled medical records of women meeting the following criteria:

2.1.Inclusion criteria

- Patients investigated for infertility who have undergone HSG and HSC,
- Spouse's spermogram compatible with intrauterine insemination.

2.2.Non inclusion criteria

- Interval of more than 3 months between the HSC and the HSG.

2.3.Exclusion criteria

- Data missing from the medical file

3. EXPLORATIONS

3.1.Procedure for hysterosalpingography

The HSG was performed on an outpatient basis. The cervix was exposed with a speculum and held with Pozzi forceps. A flexible cannula was gently inserted through the cervical canal into the uterine cavity, beyond the internal cervical os. A water-soluble, non-irritating, low osmolar, radiopaque contrast medium of approximately 10 ml was slowly injected by attaching the loaded syringe to the cannula. X-rays were then taken under fluoroscopic control and the uterine cavity and fallopian tubes were visualised. HSG was performed in all women under aseptic conditions. Instruments were removed. The women were observed for a period of time.

3.2.Procedure for hysteroscopy

HSC was performed in the operating theatre after patient consent under spinal anaesthesia during the immediate post-menstrual phase. The size and position of the uterus were confirmed physical examination and pelvic ultrasound prior to the procedure. The distension fluid was isotonic saline. In the event of any abnormality, appropriate therapeutic measures were taken.

4. COLLECTION OF DATA

Patients were registered on the basis of admission records. The data for our study were collected from medical observation records, respecting the anonymity of the patients.

4.1. Characteristics of the population studied

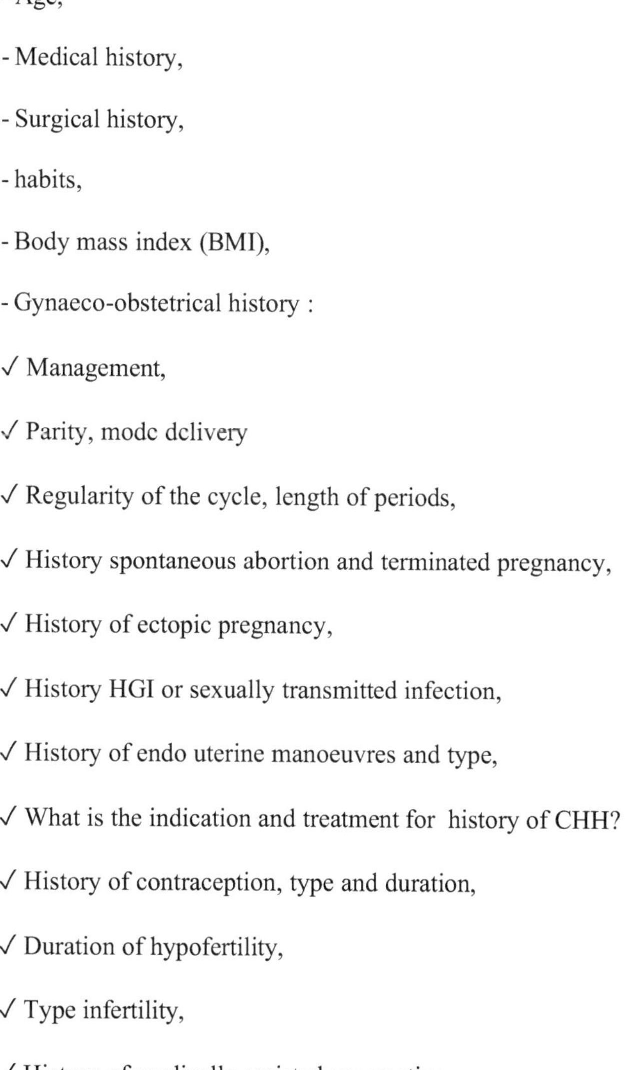

- Age,
- Medical history,
- Surgical history,
- habits,
- Body mass index (BMI),
- Gynaeco-obstetrical history :

✓ Management,

✓ Parity, modc dclivery

✓ Regularity of the cycle, length of periods,

✓ History spontaneous abortion and terminated pregnancy,

✓ History of ectopic pregnancy,

✓ History HGI or sexually transmitted infection,

✓ History of endo uterine manoeuvres and type,

✓ What is the indication and treatment for history of CHH?

✓ History of contraception, type and duration,

✓ Duration of hypofertility,

✓ Type infertility,

✓ History of medically assisted procreation.

4.2. Data from hysterosalpingography

- The day of the cycle when it is carried out,

- Size of the uterine cavity,

- In case intrauterine anomalies :

✓ Type fault,

✓ Diagnosis suspected HSG.

- Aspect of the cervico-isthmic outlet,

- The permeability of the fallopian tubes and, if there is an anomaly, specify:

✓ Type (proximal or distal),

✓ Unilateral or bilateral involvement.

- Aspect of peritoneal mixing.

4.3. Data from hysteroscopy

- The day of the cycle when it is carried out,

- Size of the uterine cavity,

- Aspect of the endometrium,

- In case intrauterine anomalies :

✓ Type fault,

✓ Diagnosis suspected by the HSC,

- Aspect of the cervico-isthmic outlet,

- The appearance of the ostia,

- Therapeutic measures taken.

5. JUDGING CRITERIA

- The HSG is considered normal in cases of

✓ Normal size and permeability of the uterine cavity (from the cervix to the uterine fundus),

✓ Absence of signs tubal occlusion of any type with a normal contour of the fallopian tubes,

✓ Normal peritoneal mixing of contrast medium.

- The criteria for a normal HSC were :

✓ A normal uterine cavity (normal shape and size, regular contours, no masses),

✓ An endometrium of normal appearance and thickness,

✓ Two ostia seen normal.

6. ANALYSIS STATISTICS

Given the lack of recent data on the prevalence of infertility in Tunisia. We used the global infertility rate estimated by the WHO for 2023 at 17.5% (2). The sample size was calculated using OpenEpi software version 3.01. Using a confidence level of 95% and an alpha risk of error of 5%, the sample size was calculated as 222 patients.All the HSGs and HSCs were carried out by specific but different people in order to reduce the risk of inter-observer bias. The data collected was analysed using IBM SPSS version 26 software, while EXCEL was used to organise the data in the form of graphs and tables.

6.1. Descriptive study

Qualitative variables were described in terms of observed numbers and frequencies.For quantitative variables, the distribution of the data was studied using skewness and kurtosis coefficients and normality tests. These variables were described by means and standard deviation in the case of a normal distribution, and by medians and interquartile ranges in the opposite case.

6.2. Analytical study

To analyse the association between two qualitative variables, we used Pearson's chi2 test to compare two frequencies where We used the Student's t test to compare two means. We used Student's t test to compare two means. degree of agreement between the two explorations was studied using the Kappa coefficient.A diagnostic test was used to determine the sensitivity, specificity, positive predictive value (PPV) and negative predictive value (NPV) of HSG compared with hysteroscopy. We used the significance threshold for $p \leq 5\%$.

7. CONSIDERATION ETHICS

In order to carry out our investigation, we requested authorisation from the head of department to access the medical records. To ensure the ethical integrity of the study, anonymity was respected during data collection and no information was collected that could be traced back to their identity.

8. RESEARCH SUPPORT BIBLIOGRAPHY

We referred to the Pubmed, Science Direct and Em-Consult databases. Our bibliographic search on these sites was carried out using combinations of the following keywords in French and English: "concordance entre hystérosalpingographie et hystéroscopie", "correlation between hysterosalpingography and hysteroscopy", "Diagnostic Value of hysterosalpingography and hysteroscopy", "methods of uterine cavity assessment".This search was completed by a cascading bibliography looking for articles cited by the authors of previous works.

A total of 234 women investigated for primary or secondary infertility were studied. Of these, 6 patients were eliminated because of an interval of more than 3 months between HSG and HSC and 6 patients because of missing data in the medical records. A total of 222 patients were included in the study (Figure 1).

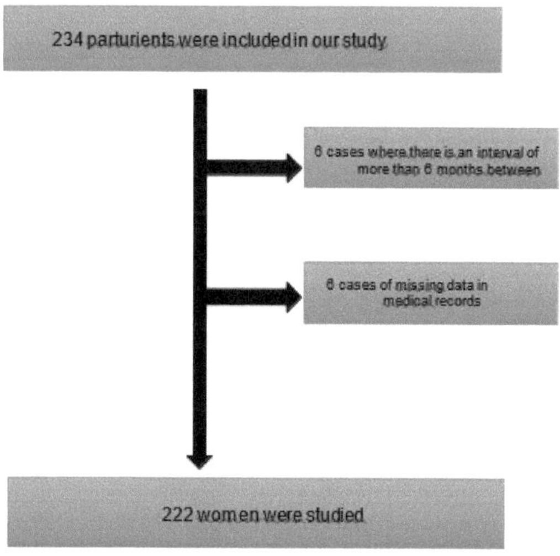

Figure 1: Flowchart of the study population.

PART I

DESCRIPTIVE STUDY

1. CHARACTERISTICS OF THE STUDY POPULATION

1.1. Age

The mean age of the women included was 35.7 years (±5.7) with extremes ranging from 21 to 45 years. The most common age was 35 to 40 years (Figure 2).

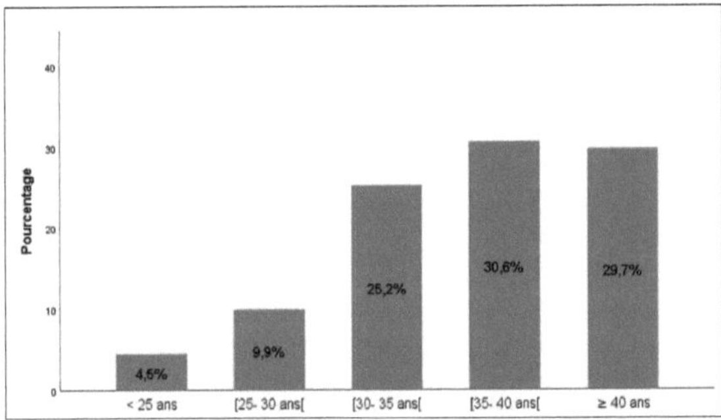

Figure 2: Age of the study population.

1.2. Medical and surgical history

1.2.1. Medical history

In the study population, 11.7% of the women included had a medical history (table I).

Table I: Summary of the medical history of the study population.

History	Workforce	Percentage (%)
Hypothyroidism	5	2,2
Polycystic ovary syndrome	5	2,2
Asthma	4	1,8
Type 2 diabetes	4	1,8
Hypertension	3	1,4
Peptic ulcer	2	0,9
Hepatitis B	2	0,9
Myasthenia	1	0,5
TOTAL	26	11,7

1.2.2. Surgical history

In the study population, 16.7% of the women included had a history of surgery, 11.7% of which was gynaecological and 5% non-gynecological (Table II).

Table II: Summary of non-gynecological surgical history in the study population.

History	Workforce	Percentage (%)
Appendectomy	7	3,2
Operated on for fracture	2	0,9
Cholecystectomy	2	0,9
TOTAL	37	16,7

KO: ovarian cyst

1.3.Habits

In the study population, the habits were :

- A smoking at 10 patients (4,5%).The average consumption was 7 pack-years.
- Alcohol consumption by two women (0.9%).
- No cases of drug addiction.

1.4. Body mass index

mean Body Mass Index (BMI) was 25.9± 3.8 Kg/m^2 with extremes of 19 to 39 Kg/m^2. The most common BMI category was normal weight (52%) (Figure 3).

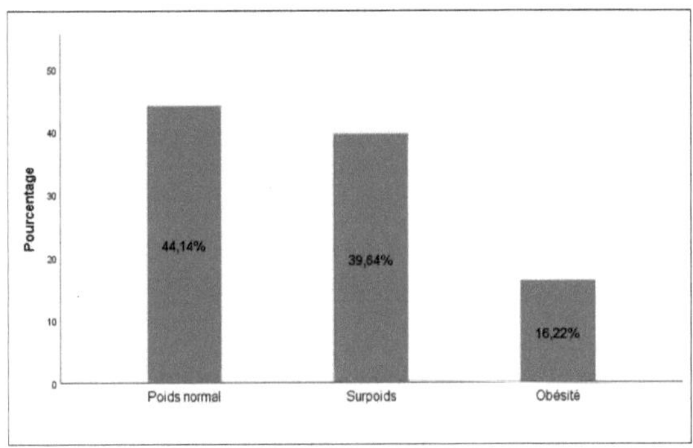

Figure 3: Distribution of the study population according BMI.

1.5. Gynaecological history and obstetrics

1.5.1. Gestité

Nulligent women represented 59.5% of the population (Figure 4).

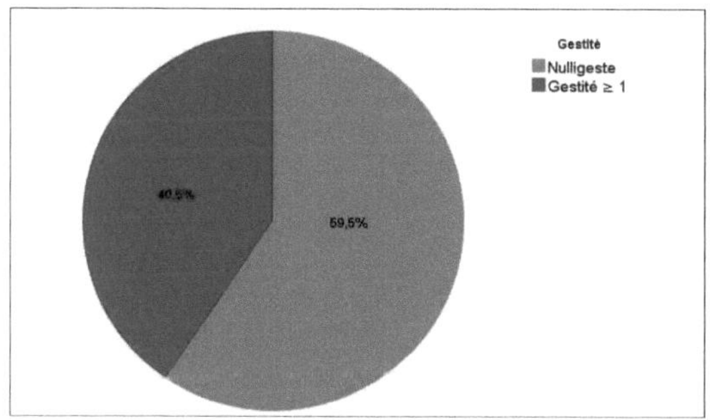

Figure 4: Distribution of women included according to gender.

1.5.2. Parity

Parity ranged from 0 to 3. Nulliparous patients accounted for 74.3% (Figure 5).

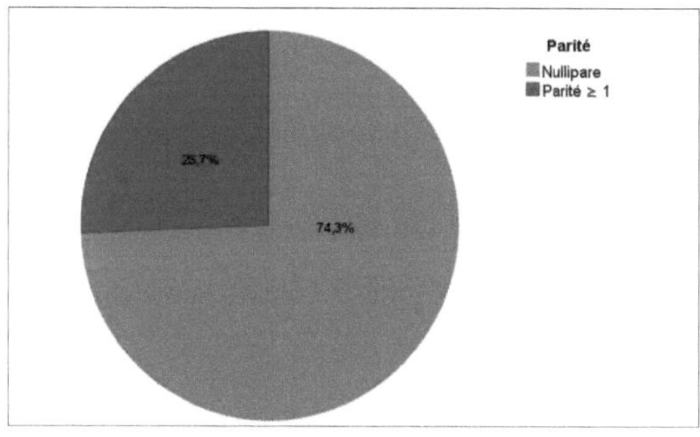

Figure 5: Gender distribution of the study population.

1.5.3. History of gynaecological surgery

In the study population, 11.7% of women had undergone surgery for a gynaecological pathology (table III).

Table III: Summary of gynaecological surgical history in the study population.

History	Workforce	Percentage (%)
Operated on for KO	10	4,5
Salpingectomy	8	3,6
Myomectomy	4	1,8
Tubal plasty	4	1,8

1.5.4. Characteristics of previous pregnancies

- A history of spontaneous abortion was noted in 38 patients (17.1%).

- A history of aborted pregnancy was noted in 17 patients (7.7%).

- A history of elective termination of pregnancy was noted two patients.

- A history of ectopic pregnancy was noted in 12 patients (5.4%). These included:

✓ Eight patients were treated by salpingectomy,

✓ Four patients were treated medically (with methotrexate).

- Among patients who had given birth previously, 55.4% had given birth vaginally and 44.6% by caesarean section. Overall, 11.3% of patients had a previous caesarean section (Figure 6).

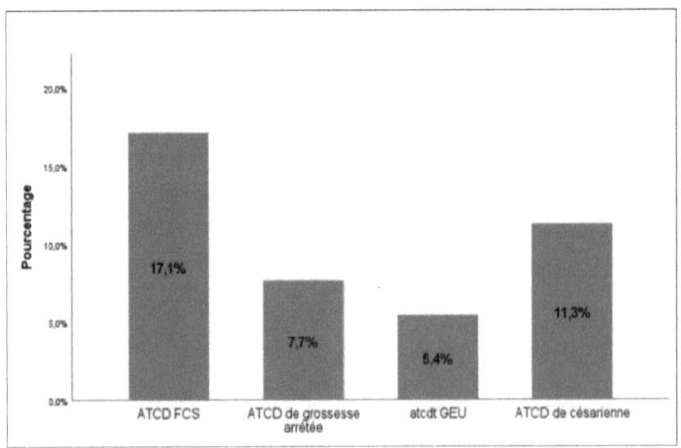

Figure 6: Percentage of characteristics of previous pregnancies.

ATCD: past history; EP: ectopic pregnancy.

1.5.5. History of gynaecological pathologies

- The menstrual cycle was regular in 93.2% of patients and irregular in 6.8% (n=15). Eight patients had spaniomenorrhoea and 7 patients had short cycles of less than 25 days.
- The average duration of blood flow was 5.5 days and only 3 women had menorrhagia.
- Of the study population, only 13 had symptoms. These included menometrorrhagia in 6 patients, dysmenorrhoea in 4 patients and dyspareunia associated with chronic pelvic pain in three patients.
- A history of upper genital infection (UGI) was noted in 7 women (3.2%).
- A history of an upper genital infection (UGI) was noted in 3 women.

- A history of endo-uterine manoeuvres in 38 women, a percentage of 17.1%. This was a

✓ Aspiration in 28 women (12.6%),

✓ HSC in ten women (4.5%) (Table IV).

Table IV: Summary of history of gynaecological pathologies.

History	Workforce	Percentage (%)
Endo uterine	38	17,1
Irregular cycle	15	6,8
IGH	7	3,2
Menometrorrhagia	6	2,7
Dysmenorrhoea	4	1,8
Dyspareunia and pain chronic pelvic pain	3	1,4
STI	3	1,4

1.5.6. Contraception

In the study population, 10.4% of women had a history of contraception. Hormonal contraception was used by 5.4% of women and intrauterine devices by 5% (Figure 7).

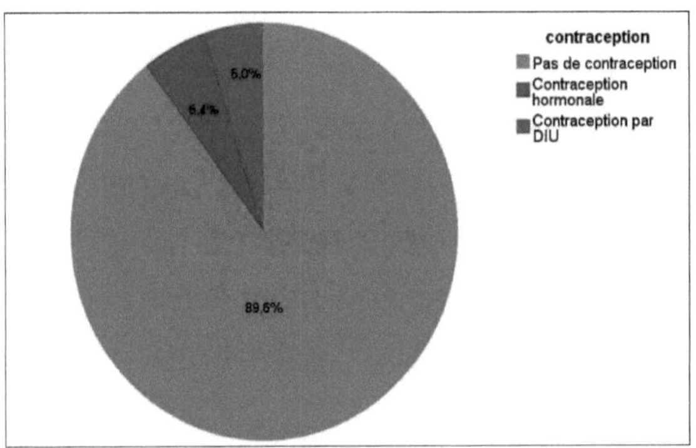

Figure 7: Summary of contraception percentages.

1.5.5. Characteristics infertility

- The majority of women, 59%, had primary infertility (n=131) and 41% had secondary infertility (n=91) (Figure 8).

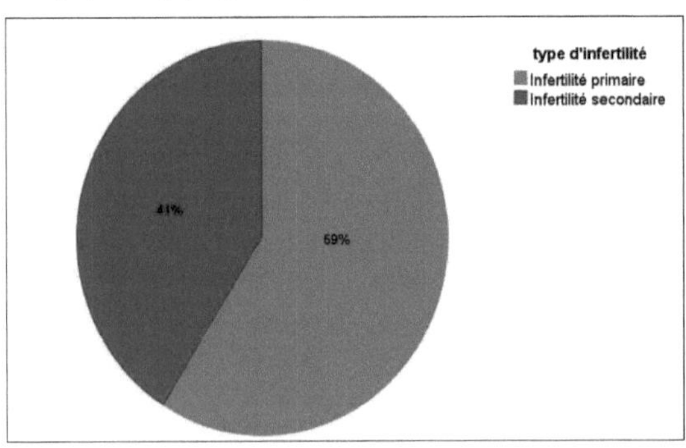

Figure 8: Percentage of types infertility.

- The duration of infertility varied between 1 and 16 years, with a median of 3 years (IQR= [2-5]).
- A hormonal work-up including measurement thyroid-stimulating hormone (TSH), prolactin, FSH, LH and oestradiol levels was performed in 90.1% of women. There were no abnormalities in any of the patients included in the study.
- The spouse's spermogram was carried out in all cases and was compatible with intrauterine insemination in all cases.
- Previous recourse to medically assisted procreation was noted 12 patients (5.4%). These were :

✓ In Vitro Fertilisation (IVF) in 6 patients,

✓ Artificial insemination with spousal sperm in 2 patients,

✓ Simple stimulation in two patients,

✓ Intracytoplasmic sperm injection in 2 patients.

2. DATA FROM HYSTEROSALPINGOGRAPHY

2.1.Day of cycle

The HSG was performed on average at day 9 ±1.5 days [5-14].

2.2.Size of the cavity

The uterine cavity was of normal size in 193 cases (86.9%) and reduced in 29 cases (13.1%).

2.3.Intra uterine anomaly cavitary

At the HSG, 87 cases of intrauterine anomalies were found (38.7%). There were no intrauterine anomalies in 135 women (61.3%) (Figure 9).In the case of abnormalities, this was an image of radiological subtraction which evoked :

✓ A polyp in 42 cases (18.9%).

✓ Synechia in 23 cases (10.4%).

✓ A myoma in 16 cases (7.2%).

✓ A malformation in 4 cases (1.8%). These were four cases of incomplete uterine septum.

✓ Only one case of isthmocoele (0.5%).

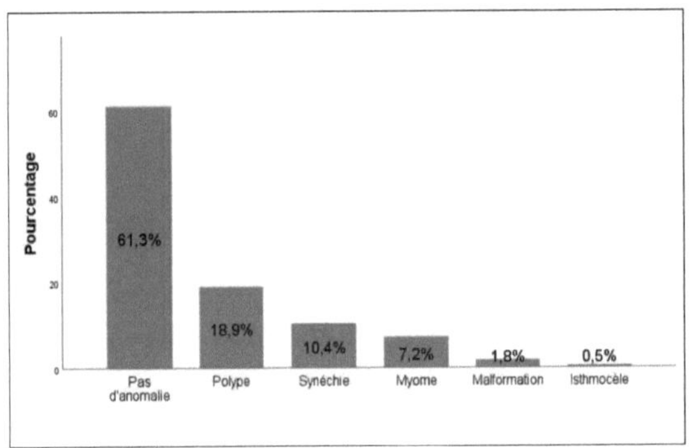

Figure 9: Percentage of intra-cavitary uterine anomalies at HSG

2.4. Cervico- isthmic defilement

Intracavitary anomalies involved the cervico-isthmic outlet in 5% of cases.

2.5. Tubal abnormalities

- There were no tubal abnormalities at HSG in 133 patients (59.8%) (Figure 10).
- Tubal anomalies were discovered by HSG in 89 patients (40.1%).

- These anomalies were unilateral in 49.4% of cases and bilateral in 50.6%.

- Their types were:

✓ An obstruction in 87.6% of cases (n=78).

✓ Hydrosalpinx with patent fallopian tubes in 12.4% of cases (n=11).

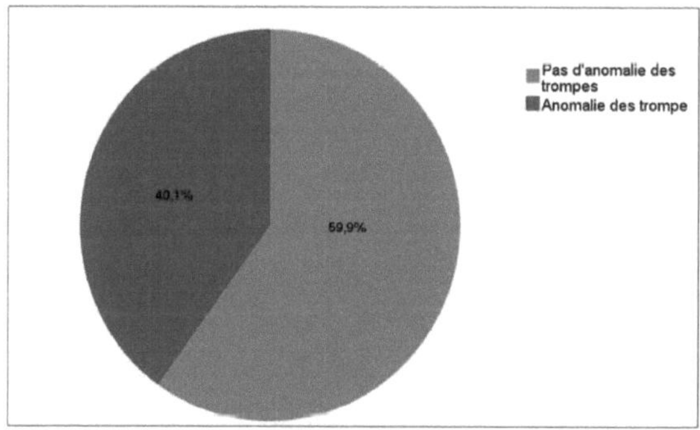

Figure 10: Percentage of types anomaly suspected HSG.

2.6. Mixing peritoneal

Peritoneal mixing was abnormal in 11 cases (5%).

3. DATA FROM HYSTEROSCOPY

3.1.Day of production cycle l'HSC

The HSG was performed on average at day 8 ±1.4 [6-13].

3.2.Size of the uterine cavity

The uterine cavity was of normal size in 183 cases (82.4%) and reduced in 39 cases (17.6%).

3.3. Aspect of the endometrium

The different aspects of the endometrium discovered at HSC are summarised in Figure 11.

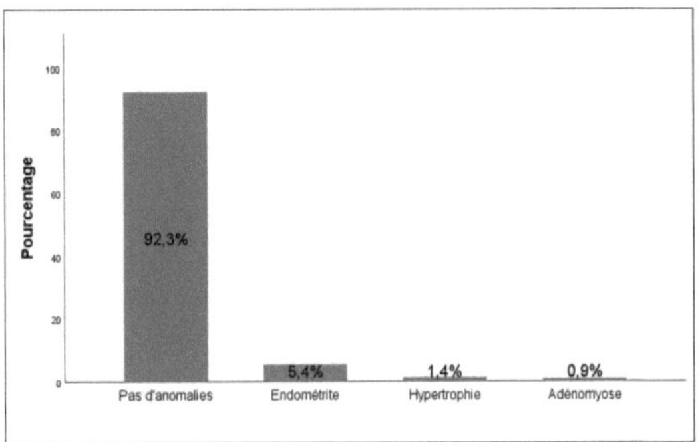

Figure 11: Percentage of endometrial anomaly at HSC.

3.4. Intrauterine anomalies

At the HSG, 92 cases of intrauterine anomalies (41.4) were discovered (Figure 12). These were :

✓ A polyp in 39 cases (17.6%).

✓ Synechia in 27 cases (12.2%).

✓ A myoma in 20 cases (9%).

✓ A malformation in 5 cases (2.3%). There were four cases of incomplete uterine septum.

✓ Only one case of isthmocoele (0.5%).

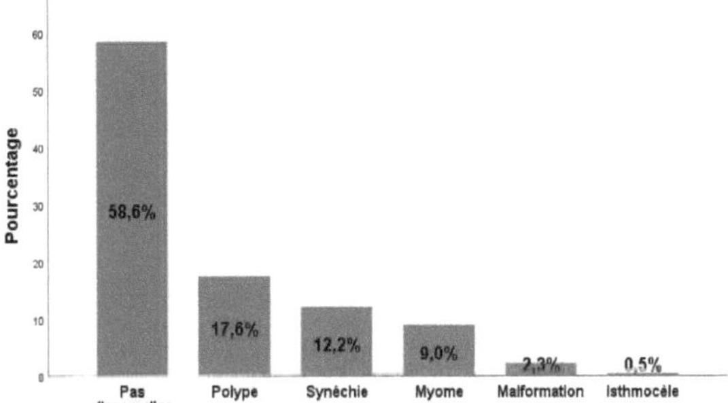

Figure 12: Percentage of intra-cavitary uterine anomalies at HSC.

3.5. Aspect of the cervico- isthmic outlet

Intracavitary anomalies involved the cervico-isthmic outlet in 5% of cases.

3.6. Aspect of ostiums

The ostia were normal except in 5 cases where they were cloudy.

3.7. Therapeutic measures

When a cavity anomaly was diagnosed, a specific procedure was performed for each lesion. These measures are summarised in Figure 13.

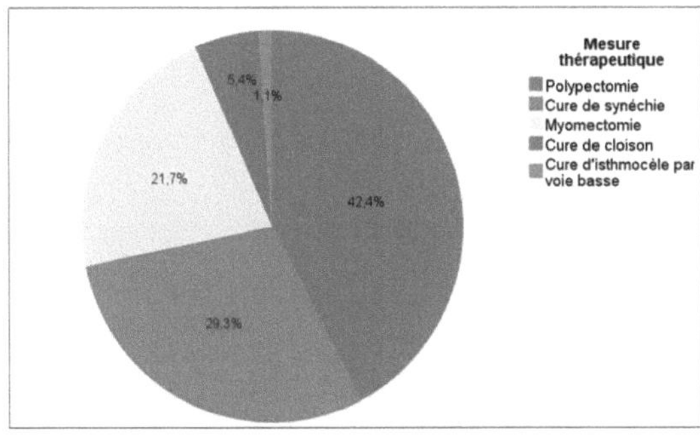

Figure 13: Percentage of therapeutic measures carried out diagnostic hysteroscopy.

PART II

ANALYTICAL STUDY

1. GOBAL COMPARISON HSG AND HSC

Taking the HSC as the reference test, we determined :

- 71 cases of uterine anomalies confirmed by HSC, i.e. 32% (true positives).

- 16 cases of abnormalities suspected on HSG but not on HSC, i.e. 7.2% (false positives).

- 114 cases of absence abnormalities HSG and HSC, i.e. 51.4% (true negatives).

- 21 cases of intra-cavitary uterine anomalies not diagnosed by HSG but discovered at HSC, i.e. 9.5% (false negative) (figure 15). These were the following anomalies:

✓ 11 cases of intracavitary polyps (5%).

✓ 8 cases of synechia (3.6%).

✓ 2 cases of intracavitary myomas (0.9%).

The following parameters for the effectiveness of HSG compared with HSC were therefore calculated:

- Sensitivity of 77.1%.

- 87.7% specificity.

- A positive predictive value (PPV) of 81.6%.

- A negative predictive value (NPV) of 84.4%.

- Positive likelihood ratio of 6.2.

- Negative likelihood ratio of 0.26.

There was an overall agreement of 83.3% between the HSG and the HSC. Comparing the two examinations, there was a statistically significant difference between them with $p<0.001$. The Kappa concordance statistical test between the 2 examinations for intra-cavitary uterine anomalies was 0.654, indicating strong agreement (table V).

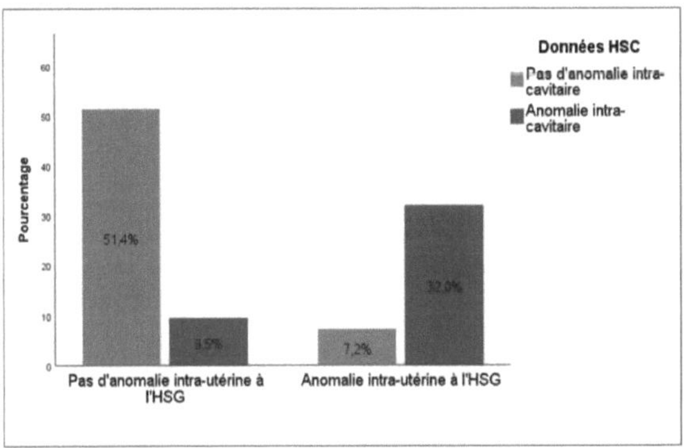

Figure 14: Distribution of results for uterine intra-cavity anomalies on HSG according to those on HSC.

Table V: Comparison of intra-cavity uterine anomalies HSG and HSC.

		Pas d'anomalies à l'HSC	Anomalies à l'HSC	P	Kappa
Anomalie à l'HSG	Non	114(84,4%)	21(15,6%)	<0,001	0,654
	Oui	16(16,4%)	71(81,6%)		

2. COMPARISON OF HSG WITH HSC ACCORDING TO TYPE OF INTRA-CAVITARY UTERINE ANOMALIES

The agreement between the two explorations according to the types of intra-cavity anomalies diagnosed was 71.3%. In fact, 62 cases of HSG abnormalities were consistent with the suspected diagnosis. Comparison of the two explorations according to lesion type showed a statistically significant difference for all lesion types and for a smaller cavity ($p<0.001$).

The kappa coefficient was 0.562 for polyps and 0.595 for synechiae, indicating moderate agreement.

This coefficient was :

- 0.817 for myomas,
- 0.887 for malformations,
- 0.792 for cavity size reduction.

This means almost perfect agreement. This means that HSG performs better for lesions such as myomas and malformations (table VI).

Table VI: Comparison and agreement between HSG and HSC according to the type of intra-cavitary uterine anomaly.

Type fault	No lesions at HSC	Presence of injury to the HSC	P	Kappa
Polyp HSG No	167(92,8%)	13(7,2%)	<0,001	0,562
Yes	16(38,1%)	26(61,9%)		
Synechia HSG No	188(94,5%)	11(5,5%)	<0,001	0,595
Yes	7(30,4%)	16(69,6%)		
Myoma at HSG No	201(97,6%)	5(2,4%)	<0,001	0,817
Yes	1(6,3%)	15(93,7%)		
malformation toNo	217(99,5%)	1(0,5%)	<0,001	0,887
HSG Yes	0(0%)	4(100%)		
Cutting cavity No	182(0,5%)	11(28,2%)	<0,001	0,792
reduced Yes	1(9,5%)	28(71,8%)		

3. COMPARISON OF HSG WITH HSC BY TYPE OF INFERTILITY

There was no significant difference between the two groups primary and secondary infertility for age, BMI and duration of infertility (table VII).

Table VII: Comparison age, BMI and duration infertility type of infertility.

Aspect	Infertility primary	Infertility secondary	P
Average age	35,5±5,6	35,8±5,7	0,683
BMI	25,5±3,7	26,3±3,7	0,147
Duration infertility	3,9±3,3	4±2,9	0,91

In our series, although cavitary anomalies were more frequent in cases of primary infertility, this difference was not statistically significant for the two investigations with p=0.513 for HSG and p=0.936 for HSC (table VIII).

Table VIII: Comparison of intra-cavitary uterine anomalies according to the type of infertility.

		Infertility primary	Infertility secondary	P
HSG abnormality	No	82(60,7%)	53(39,3%)	0,513
	Yes	49(56,3%)	38(43,7%)	
Anomaly at the HSC	No	77(59,2%)	53(40,8%)	0,936
	Yes	54(58,7%)	38(41,3%)	

The percentages of lesion types according to the type infertility are summarised in table IX.

Table IX: Percentage of lesion type according to type infertility.

		Primary infertility (%)	Secondary infertility (%)
HSG abnormalities	Polyp	24,4	11
	Synechia	4,6	18,7
	Myoma	7,6	6,6
	Malformation	0,8	3,3
	Isthmocele	0	1,1
	Total	37,4	40,7
HSC abnormalities	Polyp	41,2	41,8
	Synechia	7,6	18,7
	Myoma	9,9	7,7
	Malformation	0,8	4,4
	Isthmocele	0	1,1
	Total	41,2	41,8

The cases of malformation occurred in two women with primary infertility and 3 women with secondary infertility but history of spontaneous miscarriage.

Synechia occurred more frequently in patients with secondary infertility (18.7% vs 7.6%). This difference was statistically significant (p=0.007).

Polyps occurred more frequently in patients with primary infertility (22.9% vs 9.9%). This difference was statistically significant (p=0.002).

Myomas occurred more frequently in patients with primary infertility (9.9% vs 7.7%). This difference was not statistically significant p=0.517.

Abnormalities such as malformation and isthmocoele were more frequent in patients with secondary infertility but without any statistically significant difference (p=0.156 and p=1 respectively) (table IX).

Table X: Comparison of the types of lesions selected at the HSC according to the type of infertility.

Type fault	Infertility primary	Infertility secondary	P
Synechia	7,6%	18,7%	0,007
Polyp	22,9%	9,9	0,002
Myoma	9,9%	7,7%	0,517
Malformation	0,8%	4,4%	0,156
Isthmocele	0%	1,1%	1

Comparing the two tests in the primary and secondary infertility groups, there was a statistically significant difference between HSG and HSC ($p<0.001$). The kappa coefficient was 0.633 (Table X) and 0.684 (Table XI) respectively, which indicated strong agreement between the two groups.

Table XI: Comparison and agreement between HSG and HSC in primary infertility.

Type d'anomalie	Infertilité primaire	Infertilité secondaire	P
Synéchie	7,6%	18,7%	0,007
Polype	22,9%	9,9	0,002
Myome	9,9%	7,7%	0,517
Malformation	0,8%	4,4%	0,156
Isthmocèle	0%	1,1%	1

Table XII: Comparison and agreement between HSG and HSC in cases of secondary infertility.

		Pas d'anomalies à l'HSC	Anomalies à l'HSC	P	Kappa
Anomalie à l'HSG	Non	68(82,9%)	14(17,1%)	<0,001	0,633
	Oui	9(18,4%)	40(81,6%)		

Tableau XII : Comparaison et concordance entre l'HSG et l'HSC en cas d'infertilité secondaire.

		Pas d'anomalies à l'HSC	Anomalies à l'HSC	P	Kappa
Anomalie à l'HSG	Non	46(86,8%)	7(13,2%)	<0,001	0,684
	Oui	7(18,4%)	31(81,6%)		

DISCUSSION

Infertility is a disorder of the male or female reproductive system defined by the WHO as the inability to achieve pregnancy after 12 months or more of regular unprotected sexual intercourse (1). According to the latest estimates, it is a common condition, affecting around one in six people worldwide, with few regional differences (2). The causes of female infertility, whether primary or secondary, are divided into four pathologies: tubal, uterine, ovarian and endocrine (1). According to the literature, uterine anomalies are responsible for 10-15% of infertility. However, these anomalies can be as high as 50% in women with recurrent implantation failures (3,10). This is why assessment of the uterine cavity is part of the initial infertility . The most frequently found lesions are polyps, synechiae, myomas and uterine malformations (4).

Several imaging examinations can be used to assess the uterine cavity, including pelvic ultrasound (suprapubic and transvaginal), hydro-sonography, HSG and pelvic MRI, especially in cases of uterine malformations. Hysteroscopy can also be used, as it is the reference method for exploring the uterine cavity (10).

According to the recommendations of the French National College of Gynaecologists and Obstetricians (CNGOF) in 2022, the initial infertility should include combination of pelvic ultrasound and HSG to assess the uterine cavity. Diagnostic hysterosonography and HSC are not recommended as first-line procedures (11).

HSG is recognised as superior to trans-vaginal ultrasound for assessing the uterine cavity because of the effect of distension of the cavity during the examination that provides the best visualisation of the cavity and its permeability. Its sensitivity and specificity are better (12). HSG is an inexpensive, simple and safe examination, but it does involve radiation (6). It is also difficult to obtain in Tunisia. HSC is considered by the American Society for Reproductive Medicine to be the reference examination and the definitive method for the diagnosis and treatment of intra-cavitary uterine pathologies (13). HSC is a more invasive and more expensive method, but has the advantage of being the most effective and non-irradiating. In fact, it can diagnose subtle abnormalities that may be undetected by other tests and which may have an effect on fertility and endometrial receptivity (14).

Ambulatory HSC or HSC in the surgery is a method that is becoming increasingly popular. It is made possible by smaller hysteroscopes and improved visual systems, which make the procedure more feasible and more acceptable. This has raised the question of the indication for first-line HSC and the place of HSG in the infertility work-up (10).

In the literature, opinions are controversial as to which examination should be the first choice. Indeed, some studies consider that these two techniques are mandatory in infertility work-up. Others consider that in the case of normal HSG, HSC is no longer indicated, while other studies recommend that HSG has no place in the infertility work-up (6,9).

Another question raised is the systematic indication HSC in the assessment of unexplained infertility or prior to medically assisted procreation (15). It is therefore important to study the place of each of the two examinations in the infertility work-up and to compare their results to ensure optimal detection uterine anomalies while ensuring patient safety and security. It is within this framework that our work was integrated with the aim of :

- Comparing HSG data with HSC data in patients investigated for infertility
- Compare the performance of the two techniques in exploring the uterine cavity.

This was a retrospective, longitudinal, monocentric and comparative study carried out in department B of obstetrics and gynaecology at Charles Nicolle Hospital in Tunis, extending over 7 years and 10 months, from 1 January 2016 to 31 October 2024, and including patients being monitored for infertility who had undergone HSG and HSC.

During the study period, 222 women were included.

The most common age group between 35 and 40 (30.6%).

The majority of women, 59%, had primary infertility (n=131) and 41% had secondary infertility (n=91).

The median duration infertility was 3 years (IQR= [2-5]).

At the HSG, 87 cases of intrauterine anomalies were found (39.2%). There were no abnormalities in 135 women (60.8%). These were polyps in 48.8% of cases, synechia in 26.7% of cases, myomas in 18.6% of cases, malformations in 4.7% of , and a single case of isthmocoele. The uterine cavity was reduced in size in 13.1% of cases. Intracavitary anomalies concerned the cervico-isthmian canal in 5% of cases. Tubal anomalies were present at HSG in 89 patients (40.1%). These anomalies were bilateral in 50.6% of cases. They were obstructive in 87.6% of , and of hydrosalpinx type in 12.4% of cases.

At the HSC, 92 cases of intrauterine anomalies were discovered (41.4%). There were no anomalies in 130 women (41.4%). In the case anomaliesit was a polyp in 42.4% of cases, synechia in 29.3% of cases, myoma in 21.7% of cases, malformation in 5.4% of cases and a single case of isthmocoele. The uterine cavity was reduced in size in 17.6% of cases. HSC was also used to diagnose endometritis in 12 women, endometrial hypertrophy in 3 patients and adenomyosis in 2 patients. Intracavitary abnormalities involved the cervico-isthmic canal in 5% of cases. The ostia were veiled in 5 cases. Referring to the HSC, we identified 71 cases of uterine anomalies confirmed by the HSC (i.e. 32%) and 114 cases of no anomalies at both the HSG and the HSC (i.e. 51.4%). We identified 16 cases of anomalies suspected at HSG but not present at HSC (7.2%) and 21 cases of intra-cavitary uterine anomalies at undiagnosed HSC: 11 cases of intra-cavitary polyps (5%), eight cases of synechiae (3.6%) and two cases of intra-cavitary myomas (0.9%). The sensitivity of the HSG was determined to be 77.1%, the specificity 87.7%, the PPV 81.6%, the NPV 84.4%, the positive likelihood ratio 6.2 and the negative likelihood ratio 0.26.

There was an overall agreement of 83.3% between the HSG and the HSC. Comparing the two examinations, there was a statistically significant difference between them with $p<0.001$. The Kappa concordance statistical test between the 2 examinations for intra-cavitary uterine anomalies was 0.654, indicating strong agreement.Agreement between the two explorations according to the types of intra-cavity anomalies diagnosed was lower at 71.3%. Comparison of the two explorations according to lesion type showed a statistically significant difference for all lesion types ($p<0.001$). The kappa coefficient was 0.562 for polyps and 0.595 for synechiae, indicating moderate agreement. This coefficient was 0.817 for myomas, 0.887 for malformations and 0.792 for reduction in cavity size, which means almost perfect agreement. Synechia was associated with secondary infertility and polyps with primary infertility. Myomas, malformations and isthmocoele were not associated with the type of infertility. Comparing the two investigations in the primary infertility group and in the secondary infertility group, the agreement between the HSG and the HSC was confirmed by a statistically significant difference ($p<0.001$) and a kappa coefficient of 0.633 and 0.684 respectively, indicating strong agreement in both groups.

1. LIMITATIONS AND STRENGTHS OF THE STUDY

Study strengths :

- To our knowledge, this was the first Tunisian study to investigate the correlation between HSG and HSC according to the type of lesion and the type of infertility.
- In addition, our study was carried out at a university hospital in the capital, which enabled us to establish specialised and consistent care for our patients.
- A sufficiently large sample size to enable a proper statistical study.

Limitations of the study :

- The retrospective nature of the information gathered limits us to the data already contained in the medical file.

- The monocentric nature of the study may affect the representative nature of the results.

Despite these limitations, the results of our study provide important information for understanding the role of HSG and HSC in infertility assessment and for improving management strategies.

2. PERFORMANCE OF HYSTEROSALPINGOGRAPHY

Exploration of the uterine cavity is justified in view of the high rate of intra-cavitary anomalies, which can be as high as 50% in certain cases of infertility (10). HSG is a fairly simple and safe method of assessing the uterine cavity, which has been in existence for decades. Its place should be reassessed in light of advances in HSC, which remains the reference technique. In our study, 87 cases of intrauterine anomalies were discovered at HSG (39.2%) and 92 cases of intrauterine anomalies at HSC (41.4%). The rate of HSG anomalies varies in the literature between 8.3 and 47.1%. Our results are compared with those of the literature in Table XII.

Table XII: Comparison of the percentage of cavitary anomalies on HSG with the literature.

Study	Percentage of normal uterine	cavity	Percentage of cavities abnormal uterus
Wadhwa et al (14)	77,8		22,2
Mourali et al (16)	52,9		47,1
Panda et al (17)	76,4		23,6
Vaid et al (18)	91,7		8,3
Dalfo et al (19)	47		53
Igbodike et al (9)	85,4		14,6
Our series	60,8		39,2

Referring to the HSC, it was determined that the HSG had :

- An overall sensitivity of 77.1%,
- Specificity of 87.7%,
- 81.6% PPV
- A VPN of 84.4%.

In the literature: (table XIII)

- Sensitivity ranged from 21.3% to 81.2%.
- Specificity ranged from 33.3 to 86.6%.

This significant variability could be explained by the heterogeneity of the populations studied. Indeed, in the studies which found a sensitivity of less than 40%, this was attributed to a small number of women in the study population or to the homogeneity of the women studied, such as the majority of women consulting the clinic having infertility of male origin (14,17). Other reasons The different techniques used to perform HSG, the different methods of reporting the results and the fact that HSG is performed at different times of the menstrual cycle have been mentioned in the literature as possible explanations for these variations (14). It should be noted that the retrospective study conducted in Tunisia in 2011 over 3 years and including 140 patients by Mourali et al had the most similar sensitivity and specificity to our study (16).

Table XIII: Comparison of the sensitivity, specificity, PPV and NPV of HSG in relation to the literature.

Study	Size from the stile	Sensitivity	Specific	VPP	VPN
Igbodike et al 2022 (9)	96	88,9	33,3	87,8	35,7
Wadhwa et al. 2017 (14)	108	44.8	86.6	56.5	80.2
Mourali et al. 2011 (16)	140	76,5	77,6	74,2	79,7
Panda and al. (17)	172	42,3	85,7	59,4	75
Vaid and al. 2014 (18)	78	21,3	79,4	81,5	64,9
Dalfo and al. 2004 (19)	196	81,2	80,4	78,2	91
Our series	222	77,1	87,7	81,6	84,4

2. OVERALL CORRELATION OF HYSTEROSALPINGOGRAPHY WITH HYSTEROSCOPY

HSC is recognised as the reference method for exploring the uterine cavity by several learned societies, including the International Society for Gynecologic Endoscopy and the American Society for Reproductive Medicine. Despite its more invasive nature, this is the method that enables the final diagnosis to be made, as it visualises uterine lesions directly. It also has the advantage of allowing biopsies and therapeutic measures to be taken (7,13).

In our study, an overall agreement rate of 83.3% was observed between HSG and HSC. This meant that a significant number of uterine cavity anomalies (around 16.7%) could go undetected on HSG.

By comparing our results with those in the literature, an overall agreement varying between 71.3 and 83% was noted (Table XIV).

Incidental discovery of abnormalities by HSC was observed in 9.5% of cases, and could be the cause of infertility. These included 11 cases of intra-cavity polyps (5%), 8 cases of synechiae (3.6%) and 2 cases of intra-cavity myomas (0.9%). These lesions could have a harmful effect on fertility and could easily be treated by HSC (17). These lesions therefore justified systematic recourse to HSG, especially in cases of unexplained infertility.

The other studies also found anomalies of incidental findings detected by HSC that ranged from 7.7% to 32.1% (Table XIV).

Table XIV: Comparison of overall agreement and false negatives of HSG and HSC in the literature.

Study	Global agreement	Incidental discoveries negative)	(false
Igbodike et al (9)	80,2%	-	
Wadhwa et al (14)	71,3%	15,3%	
Mourali et al (16)	83%	10,7%	
Panda et al (17)	75%	19,1%	
Vaid et al (18)	66,3%	32,1%	
Dalfo et al (19)	73%	7,7%	
Our series	83,3%	9,5%	

To better characterise the correlation between the two tests, a comparison was made using the Chi 2 test, which showed a statistically significant difference between them with $p<0.001$.The Kappa concordance statistical test between the 2 examinations for intra-cavitary uterine anomalies was 0.654, which means strong agreement. Most studies in the literature strong agreement between the two investigations, which was similar to our study (table XV).

Table XV: Comparison of p-value and correlation coefficient with the literature.

Study	p-value	Coefficient correlation	from	Interpretation
Igbodike et al (9)	0,025	-		
Wadhwa and al. (14)	0,001	Kappa=0,336		Weak agreement
Mourali et al (16)	0,001	Q coefficient Yule= 0.83	from	Strong agreement
Panda et al (17)	<0,001	Kappa=0.74		Strong agreement
Our series	<0,001	Kappa=0,654		Strong agreement

Thus, the degree of agreement between HSG and HSC was a controversial issue in the literature. In fact, several factors are involved in infertility which may influence the different degrees of agreement reported in the literature. The time interval between the two examinations could be at the origin of the discrepancy in the discovery of uterine anomalies. It has been shown that the longer the interval, the lower the concordance due to new lesions or spontaneous involution of certain types of lesion (16).There was also inter- and intra-observer variability, indicating a degree of subjectivity in the interpretation of HSG images. One study found that this variability was low in cases of normal HSG and more pronounced in cases of abnormalities. For this reason, some authors have suggested that an exhaustive grid should be completed to minimise discrepancies in interpretation (20). Nowadays, HSC is more accessible, especially with the widespread use of outpatient HSC. This is a less invasive option given the absence of the anaesthetic risk. A recent meta-analysis in 2024 looked at the impact ambulatory HSC prior to assisted reproduction on the number of pregnancies and live births. It was concluded that ambulatory HSC increased these parameters thanks to the detection of subtle uterine intra-cavity anomalies that were not diagnosed by HSG (10).In our series, all HSCs were performed in hospital under spinal anaesthesia and, in the event of contraindications, under general anaesthesia. Another aspect to consider is the appearance of the endometrium, which is only visible on HSC. In our study, HSC diagnosed 12 cases of endometritis and two cases of adenomyosis. HSC can diagnose endometritis which has been shown to be associated with infertility (21). Treatment of chronic endometritis is associated with better IVF outcomes in patients with recurrent implantation failure (22).

To sum up, there are two opinions to consider:

- The first is the point of view adopted by the majority of learned societies who consider that HSG, being less invasive, should be indicated in the first instance to eliminate the most significant uterine anomalies which may explain the infertility. In this context, HSC is indicated as a second-line procedure in the event of an abnormal HSG.

- The second point of view is that which advocates the use of HSC as a first-line procedure in order to definitively compensate for the uterine cavity, or to confirm that a uterine anomaly is the cause of infertility and to allow treatment. This is a radical approach that is currently defended by the availability of outpatient HSCs. However, the question remains: are lesions that are invisible on HSG responsible for infertility? On the other hand, the risks incurred during of HSC, are they outweighed by the diagnostic and therapeutic advantages?

3. CORRELATION OF HYSTEROSALPINGOGRAPHY AND HYSTEROSCOPY ACCORDING TO THE TYPE OF SUSPECTED INTRA-CAVITARY UTERINE ANOMALY

After the overall comparison and to better understand the correlation between HSG and HSC, we need to specify the differences in each group of intra-cavitary uterine lesions diagnosed. Table XVI summarises the various anomalies observed in our series during the 2 examinations with those in the literature:

Table XVI: Comparison of the percentages of intrauterine anomalies in relation to the literature.

Type fault	Preutthipan et al	Mourali et al.	Our study
	HSG/HSC	HSG/HSC	HSG/HSC
Polyp	21,4% /16,7%	4% /14%	18,9% /17,6%
Synechia	41,1% /22%	6% /12%	10,4% /12,2%
Myoma	14,9% /7,7%	14% /6%	7,2% /9%)
Malformation	7,7% /5,4%	8% /5%	1,8% /2,3%

The agreement between the two explorations according to the type of intra-cavity anomaly diagnosed was 71.3%. This was lower than the overall rate. This was This is explained by the fact that HSC has the advantage of direct visualisation of the lesion.Comparison of the two explorations according to lesion type showed a statistically significant difference for all lesion types ($p<0.001$). The kappa coefficient was 0.562 for polyps and 0.595 for synechiae, indicating moderate agreement. The coefficient was 0.817 for myomas and 0.887 for malformations, indicating almost perfect agreement. In the literature, few studies have compared HSG and HSC according to the nature of the suspected intrauterine lesion. The data in the literature concurred on the fact that the diagnostic accuracy was lower if the two examinations were compared according to the type of lesion (9). This hypothesis was adopted by some authors who did not decide on a diagnosis on the basis of HSG data alone, and instead were content to describe abnormalities radiologically in three types: failure to fill the cavity, irregular cavity and small cavity (14,17). However, this approach oversimplifies the problem, since cavity filling defects take several radiological forms that could be suggestive of certain diagnoses.

4. OVERALL CORRELATION OF HYSTEROSALPINGOGRAPHY WITH HYSTEROSCOPY ACCORDING TO THE TYPE OF INFERTILITY

In our series, the rate primary infertility was 59% and secondary 41%. These rates were comparable to those found in the literature (table XVII).

Table XVII: Comparison of primary and secondary infertility rates with those in the literature.

Study	Percentage primary infertility	Percentage secondary infertility
Igbodike et al (9)	64%	36%
Wadhwa et al (14)	74%	26%
Mourali et al (16)	58%	42%
Panda et al (17)	65%	35%
Vaid et al (18)	66%	34%
Our series	59%	41%

In our study, there was no significant difference between the two groups of primary and secondary infertility for age, BMI and duration of infertility. This was in line with the literature except for age, which was generally higher in secondary infertility (14).In our series, although cavitary anomalies were more frequent in cases of primary infertility, this difference was not statistically significant for the two investigations with p=0.513 for HSG and p=0.936 for HSC. This was in line with the literature (14).

Synechia was associated secondary infertility and polyps with primary infertility. Myomas, malformations and isthmocoele were not associated with the type of infertility. In the literature, synechiae were more frequent in patients with secondary infertility. Polyps and myomas were not associated with any type infertility. Malformations were more likely to be diagnosed in women with primary infertility (16).In our study, malformations occurred predominantly in patients with secondary infertility. This could be explained by the fact the malformations discovered were all of the incomplete uterine septum type, which was more likely to be a cause of recurrent miscarriage.Comparing the two investigations in the primary infertility group and the secondary infertility group, the agreement between the HSG and the HSC was confirmed by a statistically significant difference ($p<0.001$) and a kappa coefficient of 0.633 and 0.684 respectively, indicating strong agreement in both groups. In the literature, there was no comparison between the two explorations according to the type of infertility.

5. RECOMMENDATIONS

Our work has highlighted the importance of comparing HSG and HSC, and of discussing the place of each of the two investigations in ensuring that patients being monitored for infertility receive the best possible care. Taking into account the advantages of each, our results and current international recommendations, we have made the following recommendations:

- Given its sensitivity and specificity in our study and in the literature, and the strong agreement with HSC, hysterography remains a recommended first-line examination. It is simple and inexpensive to perform, and also allows assessment of the uterine cavity, the state of the fallopian tubes and the peritoneal cavity. It also provides a document that can be reassessed by the various specialists treating the patient.

- If there is an abnormality on HSG, HSC is clearly indicated, as it is the reference technique that makes the final diagnosis and enables treatment to be carried out.
- The benefits of HSC in cases normal HSG are still controversial. Based on the current state of the literature and on our data, it is impossible to make a recommendation for systematic HSC. However, in the case of normal HSG, there is evidence in the literature of the value of the indication of an HSC prior to a planned medically assisted procreation technique such as IVF. In other cases there is no evidence.

CONCLUSIONS

Abnormalities of the uterine cavity are frequent causes of female infertility, accounting for between 10 and 15% of all causes of infertility. The most common lesions include polyps, synechiaemyomas and uterine malformations.
According to current recommendations, the uterine cavity is studied using a combination of pelvic ultrasound and HSG. If an abnormality is suspected on these two examinations, an HSC is recommended. HSC is the reference method for assessing the uterine cavity, enabling diagnostic confirmation and therapeutic intervention. HSG is a simple, inexpensive and safe method which still has an important place in the first-line assessment and determines subsequent management. However, there is controversy between authors. Some authors suggest that HSC is a compulsory examination in the investigation of infertility since HSC is the gold standard and since some cases of intra-cavity anomalies may be invisible HSG. Other authors consider that HSC is only indicated in cases of abnormalities on HSG, as HSG is a less invasive, more accepted and safer technique.It is therefore essential to compare the two tests in order to determine the role of each in the infertility assessment.
It is within this framework that our study was carried out with the aim of :

- Comparing HSG data with HSC data in patients investigated for infertility
- Compare the performance of the two techniques in exploring the uterine cavity.

This was a retrospective, longitudinal, monocentric and comparative study carried out in Department B of Obstetrics and Gynaecology Charles Nicolle Hospital in Tunis, spanning 7 years and 10 months, from 1 January 2016. until 31 October 2024, including patients being monitored for infertility who have undergone HSG and HSC.

During the study period, 222 women were included. The most common age group between 35 and 40 (30.6%). The majority of women, 59%, had primary infertility (n=131) and 41% of women had secondary infertility (n=91) with a median duration of infertility of 3 years (IQR= [2-5]).

- At the HSG, 87 cases of intrauterine anomalies were discovered (39.2%). These included polyps in 48.8% of cases, synechia in 26.7%, myomas in 18.6%, malformations in 4.7%, and a single case of isthmocoele. The uterine cavity was reduced in size in 13.1% of cases.
- At the HSC, 92 cases intrauterine anomalies were discovered (41.4%). Abnormalities included polyps in 42.4% of cases, synechia in 29.3% of , myomas in 21.7% of , malformations in 5.4% of cases and a single case of isthmocoele. The uterine cavity was reduced in size in 17.6% of cases. HSC was also used to diagnose endometritis in 12 women, endometrial hypertrophy in three and adenomyosis in two.

Referring to the HSC, we identified 71 cases of uterine anomalies confirmed by the HSC (i.e. 32%) and 114 cases of no anomalies at both the HSG and the HSC (i.e. 51.4%). We identified 16 cases of anomalies suspected at HSG but not present at HSC (7.2%) and 21 cases of intra-cavitary uterine anomalies at undiagnosed HSC: 11 cases of intra-cavitary polyps (5%), eight cases of synechiae (3.6%) and two cases of intra-cavitary myomas (0.9%).

The sensitivity of the HSG was determined to be 77.1%, the specificity 87.7%, the PPV 81.6%, the NPV 84.4%, the positive likelihood ratio 6.2 and the negative likelihood ratio 0.26. There was an overall agreement of 83.3% between the HSG and the HSC. Comparing the two examinations, there was a statistically significant difference ($p<0.001$). The Kappa concordance test between the 2 examinations for intra-cavitary uterine anomalies was 0.654, indicating strong agreement. Agreement between the two explorations according to the type of intra-cavity anomalies diagnosed was lower at 71.3%. Comparison of the two investigations according to lesion type showed a statistically significant difference for all lesion types ($p<0.001$). The kappa coefficient was 0.562 for polyps and 0.595 for synechiae, indicating moderate agreement. The coefficient was 0.817 for myomas, 0.887 for malformations and 0.792 for reduction in cavity size, indicating almost perfect agreement.

Comparing the two investigations in the primary infertility group and the secondary infertility group, there was a statistically significant difference ($p<0.001$) and a kappa coefficient of 0.633 and 0.684 respectively, indicating strong agreement in both groups.

In conclusion, we highlighted the importance of raising awareness of the effectiveness of HSG compared with HSC by knowing the limitations and advantages of this examination in order to enable better management of infertile women. At the end of this work, it is clear that HSG retains an important place in the first-line assessment and should be indicated given its strong agreement with HSC. Furthermore, it is undeniable that HSC should be indicated when an abnormality is suspected on HSG. However, there is still some uncertainty as to whether HSC should be routinely performed if the HSG is normal. The literature reports a non-negligible rate of false negatives that will not be diagnosed at HSG and could have a negative effect on fertility. By specifying the type of population, we can make a recommendation for an HSC before resorting to medically induced pregnancy.Future larger studies should investigate the role of HSC in normal HSG in unexplained infertility and recurrent miscarriage.

REFERENCES

1. World Health Organization. infertility. May 2024;1-2.

2. Word Health Organization. 1 in 6 people globally affected by infertility. Apr 2023;1-2.

3. Pundir J, El Toukhy T. Uterine cavity assessment prior to IVF. Womens Health Lond Engl. Nov 2010;6(6):841-7; quiz 847-8.

4. Carson SA, Kallen AN. Diagnosis and Management of Infertility. JAMA. 6 Jul 2021;326(1):65-76.

5. ESHRE Add-ons working group, Lundin K, Bentzen JG, Bozdag G, Ebner T, Harper J, et al. Good practice recommendations on add-ons in reproductive medicine†. Hum Reprod Oxf Engl. 2 Nov 2023;38(11):2062-104.

6. Panda SR, Kalpana B. The Diagnostic Value of Hysterosalpingography and Hysterolaparoscopy for Evaluating Uterine Cavity and Tubal Patency in Infertile Patients. Cureus. 6 Jan 2021;13(1):e12526.

7. The International Society for Gynecologic Endoscopy. Diagnostic hysteroscopy: patient assessment and preparation. 2023;1-14.

8. Ait Benkaddour Y, Gervaise A, Fernandez H. [Which is the method of choice for evaluating uterine cavity in infertility workup?] J Gynecol Obstet Biol Reprod (Paris). Dec 2010;39(8):606-13.

9. Igbodike EP, Badejoko OO, Fasubaa OB, Ibitoye BO, Loto OM, Ikechebelu JI, et al. Correlation between hysterosalpingography diagnosis and final hysterolaparoscopy with dye-test diagnosis in women with utero-tubal infertility: A cross-sectional study of the implication for which test should be the first-line investigation. SAGE Open Med. 2022;10:20.

10. Hou JH, Lu BJ, Huang YL, Chen CH. Outpatient hysteroscopy impact on subsequent assisted reproductive technology: a systematic review and meta-analysis in patients with normal transvaginal sonography or hysterosalpingography images. Reprod Biol Endocrinol RBE. 1 Feb 2024;22(1):18.

11. Sonigo C, Robin G, Boitrelle F, Fraison E, Sermondade N, Mathieu d'Argent E, et al. First-line management of infertile couples: an update of the RPC 2010 of the CNGOF. Gynécologie Obstétrique Fertil Sénologie. 1 May 2024;52(5):305-35.

12. Devine K, Dolitsky S, Ludwin SI, Ludwin A. Modern Assessment of the Uterine Cavity and Fallopian Tubes in the Era of High-Efficacy ART. Fertil Steril. Jul 2022;118(1):19-28.

13. Practice Committee of the American Society for Reproductive Medicine. Practice Committee of the American Society for Reproductive Medicine. Fertility evaluation of infertile women: a committee opinion. Fertil Steril. Nov 2021;116(5):1255-65.

14. Wadhwa L, Rani P, Bhatia P. Comparative Prospective Study of Hysterosalpingography and Hysteroscopy in Infertile Women. J Hum Reprod Sci. 2017;10(2):73-8.

15. Kamath MS, Rikken JFW, Bosteels J. Does Laparoscopy and Hysteroscopy Have a Place in the Diagnosis of Unexplained Infertility? Semin Reprod Med. Jan 2020;38(1):29-35.

16. Mourali M, Nabil BZ, Chiraz EF. Investigation infertility: Correlation of hysterography and hysteroscopy. Tunis Med. 2011;90.

17. Panda SR, Kalpana B. The Diagnostic Value of Hysterosalpingography and Hysterolaparoscopy for Evaluating Uterine Cavity and Tubal Patency in Infertile

Patients. Cureus. 13(1):e12526.

18. Vaid K, Mehra S, Verma M, Jain S, Sharma A, Bhaskaran S. Pan endoscopic approach "hysterolaparoscopy" as an initial procedure in selected infertile women. J Clin Diagn Res JCDR. Feb 2014;8(2):95-8.

19. Roma Dalfó A, Ubeda B, Ubeda A, Monzón M, Rotger R, Ramos R, et al. Diagnostic value of hysterosalpingography in the detection of intrauterine abnormalities: a comparison with hysteroscopy. AJR Am J Roentgenol. Nov 2004;183(5):1405-9.

20. Renbaum L, Ufberg D, Sammel M, Zhou L, Jabara S, Barnhart K. Reliability of clinicians versus radiologists for detecting abnormalities on hysterosalpingogram films. Fertil Steril. Sept 2002;78(3):614-8.

21. Ticconi C, Inversetti A, Marraffa S, Campagnolo L, Arthur J, Zambella E, et al. Chronic endometritis and recurrent reproductive failure: a systematic review and meta-analysis. Front Immunol. 2024;15:1427454.

22. Vitagliano A, Saccardi C, Noventa M, Di Spiezio Sardo A, Saccone G, Cicinelli E, et al. Effects of chronic endometritis therapy on in vitro fertilization outcome in women with repeated implantation failure: a systematic review and meta-analysis. Fertil Steril. 1 Jul 2018;110(1):103- 112.e1.

APPENDICES

Pre-prepared information form

Characteristics of the population studied :

- Age in years
- Medical history
- Surgical history
- Lifestyle habits: Tobacco, alcohol, drug addiction
- BMI
- Gynaeco-obstetrical history :

✓ Gestité

✓ Parity

✓ Regularity of cycle, duration of blood flow, history of menometrorrhagia-like symptoms or pelvic pain or dysmenorrhoea or dyspareunia

✓ History of spontaneous miscarriage or terminated pregnancy

✓ History abortion

✓ History of ectopic pregnancy, treatment used

✓ History HGI or STI

✓ History of endo-uterine manoeuvres Y/N ? what type

✓ History of contraception of what type and for how long

✓ Duration hypofertility

✓ Type infertility

✓ Any history of medically assisted procreation and of what type

Data from l'HSG

✓ Day of production cycle

✓ Intrauterine anomaly, what type and diagnosis suspected HSG

✓ Size of the uterine cavity

✓ Tubal anomaly, unilateral or bilateral, what type of proximal or distal obstruction?

Data from l'HSC

✓ Day of production cycle

✓ Cavity size

✓ What type of intracavitary anomaly?

✓ Appearance of ostia

✓ Aspect of the cervico-isthmic outlet

HYSTEROSAPINGOGRAPHY VERSUS HYSTEROSCOPY IN INFERTILITY: PERFORMANCES FOR INTRA-UTERINE ANOMALIES' DIAGNOSIS

ABSTRACT

Background

Hysterosalpingography and hysteroscopy are the two tests traditionally used to explore the uterine cavity in case of infertility. However, there is controversy concerning the role and place of each examination. The aim of our study was to compare hysterosalpingography and hysteroscopy results and to determine the performance of each technique in diagnosing intrauterine anomalies in infertility.

Methods

This was a retrospective, longitudinal and descriptive study. It was conducted at the Obstetrics and Gynecology Department B of Charles Nicolle Hospital in Tunis, over a seven-year and ten months period. Patients treated for infertility who have undergone both hysterosalpingography and hysteroscopy were included.

Results

During the study period, 222 women were included. Most women (59%) had primary infertility and 41% had secondary infertility. Hysterosalpingography revealed 87 cases (39.2%) of intrauterine anomalies. Hysteroscopy revealed 92 cases (41.4%) of intrauterine anomalies. 21 cases of intra-cavitary uterine anomalies were identified by hysteroscopy and not diagnosed by hysterosalpingography (11 polyps, eight synechiae, two myomas). The sensitivity of hysterosalpingography was 77.1%, specificity 87.7%, positive predictive value 81.6%, negative predictive value 84.4%. Overall agreement between hysterosalpingography and hysteroscopy was 83.3%. There was a statistically significant difference between the two tests ($p<0.001$). The Kappa agreement test between the 2 explorations for intra-cavitary uterine anomalies *was 0.654, indicating strong agreement.*

Conclusion

Hysterosalpingography retains its place as a first-line examination in infertility assessment, since its agreement with hysteroscopy has been proven. Hysteroscopy is indicated as a second-line procedure in the event of abnormalities on hysterosalpingography. The indication for first-line hysteroscopy deserves further study.

TABLE OF CONTENTS

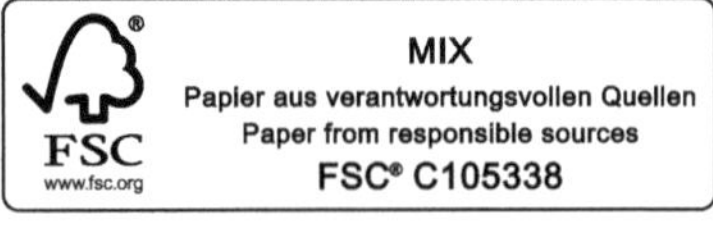

Printed by Books on Demand GmbH, Norderstedt / Germany